Cupping Therapy

An Essential Guide to Cupping Therapy, How It Works, and Its Benefits

by Anada Priso

Table of Contents

Introduction

Cupping is a medical practice where cups are placed on parts of the body to create a suction effect which raises the skin and draws the blood to the surface. It is used throughout Asia, the Middle East, and Europe to treat pain, swelling, inflammation, migraine, rheumatism, bronchitis, and the common cold. Recent studies suggest that it could also be a promising form of treatment for a host of other ailments, as well.

The earliest known use of this technique is found in the Ebers Papyrus from Egypt, which is about 5,000 years old. In China, it is mentioned in medical treatises that go back some 3,000 years. Hippocrates, the Greek doctor who composed the Hippocratic Oath, mentions it in 400 BC. The prophet Mohammad recommended the practice in the Koran 1400 years ago, while in Finland, they've been doing it since the 15th century.

Though little known here in America, this form of treatment is still popular throughout Asia, the Middle East, and Finland. As such, it is called by many names including *ba gwan, giac hoi, bekam, buhang,* and *bentusa* in Southeast Asia. In the Middle East, it is commonly referred to as *hijama*, *hejamat*, and *badkesh*, among many others.

The procedure involves using glass or ceramic cups, metal bells, bamboo tubes, animal horn, and a wide host of other items. Recently, however, the use of glass jars, plastic, and silicone are becoming more popular.

Cotton is soaked in alcohol or medicated oil and ignited. This is then put inside the container to heat it, lowering its internal pressure. The cup is immediately placed on the skin, and as the air inside cools, it creates a vacuum effect which makes it stick to the skin.

Blood immediately rushes to the area, creating a painless bruise which actually feels good. Those who have gone through the procedure claim it feels like a massage in reverse. Instead of pressure bearing down against the skin, it feels like the skin is being pushed outward, instead.

Depending on how the bruising occurs, its coloration, and how long it lasts, practitioners can tell where problems are located and can prescribe different treatments accordingly. These can range anywhere from massage, acupuncture, dietary recommendations, drug prescriptions, even to bleeding.

There are two types of cupping: wet and dry. The former involves bleeding and tends to be used more throughout Finland and the Middle East. With the exception of wet cupping, the process is generally painless and even feels relaxing.

Chapter 1: Preparing for a Session

While cupping is available in America, it qualifies as a form of alternative treatment. As such, you should be wary of some of the health claims that fans and practitioners say about it.

Some believe it can cure various forms of cancer, citing incredible medical testimonies from China, Southeast Asia, and the Middle East. As of 2014, the American Cancer Society insists that such reports are largely anecdotal and not the result of credible research findings which would pass sufficient medical scrutiny.

Cancer aside, in 1990, a peer-reviewed clinical study reported that cupping was found to be effective in treating anterior knee pain and improving range of motion. A 2012 study found that in tandem with other treatments, it was also effective in treating some cases of acne, cervical spondylosis, facial paralysis, and herpes zoster. Please note, however, that the operative words here are "some cases of" and "in tandem with other treatments."

Even practitioners generally admit that cupping's ability to heal is extremely limited. If you do have a medical condition you need treated, it's best to consult with your general practitioner first. You're also better off using tried and tested medical techniques as your primary source of treatment. It is important to understand that this book only explains cupping. It neither encourages it nor prescribes it as a viable form of therapy.

While not supporting claims that it can heal diseases, the American Medical Association considers dry cupping to be a generally safe and harmless practice. As such, a number of massage centers and spas can safely and legally offer it as a form of relaxation—even without going through the years of training that serious practitioners undergo.

In many Southeast Asian countries, cupping is offered on the sidewalks to passersby who need a quick, cheap, and effective way of easing headaches, neck and back pain, as well as joint and muscle stiffness. In Europe, cupping has even evolved into a form of vacuum massage. Instead of burning alcohol, a mechanical vacuum pump is placed on the skin and rubbed all over the body to provide exactly the type of reverse massage described in the introduction.

So the process is generally safe and it rarely hurts. If you do suffer from pain in the knees and joints, as well as some of the other conditions listed earlier, it could work for you. Some doctors suggest that those suffering from hemophilia should avoid this treatment, but in 2001, some British researchers found that it can help hemophiliacs in some cases (maybe because the entire Royal Family are hemophiliacs).

Once again, please consult with your GP first.

Chapter 2: What to Expect from a Dry Session

This is the most common type and is relatively painless unless you suffer from skin allergies, rashes, or overly sensitive skin. If you do have a dry cupping session with experts, it is usually offered as part of a larger series of treatments and is rarely used as a stand-alone form of therapy.

The procedure is usually done to your back, neck, and shoulders, but rarely on the limbs. In Chinese medicine, they take care to avoid cupping on skin ulcers or on the sacral regions of women who are pregnant.

Prior to a treatment, you may be asked to brush your teeth while taking care to avoid scraping your tongue. This is because traditional Chinese medicine uses body temperature, skin tone, heartbeat, and the appearance of your tongue as a means of assessing your state of health.

You may then be asked to remove your shirt (and if you're a woman, your bra) and made to lie on your stomach. The doctor will then burn a bit of cotton and stick it into a glass ball with an open lip on one end. This open end will be stuck to your skin, causing an immediate suction.

The burning cotton will not be kept inside the ball, so you shouldn't worry about getting burned. The cup will only be heated briefly, so the most you'll feel is a warm, round, glass being stuck on you.

You will feel the suction immediately as your flesh rises into the lip. Depending on your condition, you can expect anywhere from one to as many as ten (or more) cups getting stuck to your neck, shoulders, and back. The longer the cups are kept on, the tighter the suction becomes. Most find it pleasurable and relaxing. Hopefully, so will you.

Bony areas, like your shoulders and neck, will get smaller cups to intensify the suction and keep them on. Fleshier areas like your back will get bigger cups so they can suck in more of your skin. Silicone is used more and more for better suction on bonier sections.

Blood will then rush to the surface of your skin, causing a painless bruise, and your pores will open up. Your doctor will be watching carefully, because the extent of the coloration and other changes to the affected skin area will form part of his/her diagnosis.

According to traditional Chinese medicine, the blood will also flow better to areas that have been starved of oxygen. Chi, a power inherent in your body, will also focus on the spot to promote healing and recharge that weakened part.

Your doctor will then remove the cup after three to five minutes. Removal is also painless, after which you'll look like you've been attacked by an octopus. The darker the bruising, the more your doctor will focus upon it. A normal bruise should be a vibrant reddish or reddish orange.

It usually takes three to four days for it to leave completely, though in some cases, it can take as long as a week. This is an important thing you must take into consideration in case you're expecting to join a bathing suit contest shortly after.

If you do feel pain, you must let your doctor know right away, though this is extremely rare. In lieu of glass, some clinics prefer to use plastic or hypoallergenic silicone cups. It should be noted, however, that these other materials do not in any way mitigate the amount of bruising that results.

The area will not be tender or sore, despite the ugly coloration left behind. Normal bruising is usually caused because the area has been hit hard enough. Since no hitting is involved, it will actually look a lot worse than it feels.

A massage or acupuncture treatment may follow if you go to a traditional Chinese clinic. In cities throughout Southeast Asia where cuppers ply their trade on the streets, cupping is about all you'll get out of the session, though some may insist on giving you a backrub if they feel you need it.

Some feel a mild tingling on their skin after the cups are removed. This can last anywhere from several minutes to a couple of hours, which is normal, depending on the situation.

In cases where you're suffering from stiff joints or aching muscles, you may be asked to come in for several sessions. If so, they'll usually ask you to come back after the bruising is gone. At most, you may get two sessions in a week. Three sessions a week is not recommended, so if you get an offer for one, you're not in a traditional Chinese clinic. Most likely, you've wandered into a spa.

Since Chinese medicine believes that ill-health is the result of many factors including the accumulation of toxins in your body, you'll be asked to drink plenty of water after each cupping session. The general recommendation is about eight 8 oz glasses of water everyday throughout the course of your treatment.

Since dry cupping is usually part of a much more holistic series of treatments, an entire session can last anywhere between 15 minutes to an hour. Depending on your symptoms, your treatment can involve certain exercises, the drinking of certain teas, and even lifestyle changes like cutting down on alcohol or giving up smoking.

Other forms of treatment may also follow, which will be covered in the next chapters.

Chapter 3: Ventosa — Moving or Rubbing Cupping

In this version, medicated oil is rubbed on the skin. Once the cups are placed on the skin, the therapist will wait several minutes to maximize the suction effect. The cups will then be moved over the body, pulling up other parts of your flesh. Since the cups will inevitably pop off, they have to be heated repeatedly and replaced on the skin. After several minutes, the cups are removed and a deep tissue massage usually follows.

A modern technique involves a vacuum device placed on oiled skin. The therapist or masseur/masseuse then moves the nozzle over the shoulders, neck, and back to provide a massage. Some move the pump quickly enough to prevent the deep bruising that occurs with the traditional method. Though relaxing, this is less about treatment and more about the simple pleasure of a new massage technique.

Ventosa, using this new vacuum technology, can now also be used on the face. The use of oils and creams together with silicone pumps mitigates the bruising, and in some cases, gets rid of bruises which result from injuries. This new application of ventosa has also been found promising in the treatment of acne and facial tics.

Research is showing that ventosa with this vacuum may also be effective at finding deep tissue and muscular problems, again by observing the bruising which occurs without having to resort to surgery. Mitigating minor scars and stretch marks are other areas which seem promising as of this writing.

Others simply prefer using this new technology because, in the hands of a trained professional, they avoid the relatively long-term bruising which can result from cupping. Although some centers which offer this method claim it can also break down cellulite, no comprehensive research has yet been done on the matter as of 2015. MediCupping is a company which provides this technology, if you're interested.

Whether your cupping session involves ventosa or not, you should see to it that the cups are not kept on the same spot for more than 5 minutes. Prolonged cupping, or having a session more than twice a week, can cause capillary expansion, fluid accumulation in tissues, and even the rupture of blood vessels. Skin inflammation and the more painful Indian rope burn on the skin can also result if done excessively.

If done by a certified professional, you will never be left alone while those cups are stuck to you. If you do find yourself in a clinic where the doctor or attendant keeps leaving you to take care of other stuff, you may want to go elsewhere. Remember, one of their jobs is to observe how your skin reacts to the suction process.

Chapter 4: Cupping and Acupuncture

If you hate needles, stick to the masseurs, because cupping and needles are virtually synonymous in traditional Chinese medicine. It wasn't always so, however. According to the historical texts, cupping once stood on its own and was prescribed for chronic pulmonary diseases as it still is today.

By the time of the Tang Dynasty (AD 618–907), however, acupuncture was used to lend greater "oomph" to cupping. They would cup the patient first, then place needles on the acupuncture points, or acupoints, and finally place heated bamboo tubes over the needles to make the acupuncture work faster and deeper.

This is not practiced today, however. If you go to a traditional Chinese clinic, you'll first be assessed, and if they recommend cupping, they'll also recommend acupuncture, but not at the same time. The acupuncture session will take place after you get cupped. Since the affected area will still be bruised and tingling, the needles hurt a lot less as they go in, for some reason.

To give the needles greater penetrating power without having to push them in deeper, there's moxibustion (to be discussed later) and electricity. With the latter, the needles are attached to electrodes which deliver an electrical charge through the needles and deep into your flesh.

And yes, it hurts.

As to whether acupuncture works or not is best left up to the experts who can't seem to form a consensus on the practice. Just know that if you do have a cupping session in a traditional Chinese clinic, it will almost always be followed up by an acupuncture session.

Chapter 5: Cupping and Moxibustion

The Chinese word for moxibustion is *jiǔ* and involves heat and mugwort, as well as needles, sometimes. If you dry mugwort, age it properly, then pound it into a mold and set one end on fire, it'll burn very slowly to the other end like a cigar.

The mold is tubular and wrapped in coils of paper so that as it burns, the paper slowly flakes off like cigarette ash. Since the dried mugwort is concentrated in the middle, what's left is a sharpened point that can focus the heat while producing a medicinal smoke and scent (like incense, only less fragrant).

Depending on the symptoms and treatment, as well as the bruising that results after dry cupping, moxibustion is sometimes called for. There are three ways this is applied.

Direct scarring is done by making a small cone of dried mugwort and placing it directly on the skin. The tip is lit then blown out, allowing it to burn like incense and singe the skin till it blisters. In such cases, this is usually done after cupping (but not always) to mitigate the pain.

Direct non-scarring is the same as above, except that they remove the burning mugwort before it singes your skin.

Indirect moxibustion involves using that tubular mold like a cigar and placing its tip near various acupoints in lieu of needles. An alternative method involves puncturing your skin with acupuncture needles, then placing cones of dried mugwort atop those needles and setting them alight then blowing them out. The incense-like mugwort heats the needles, carrying that heat deep into your skin while avoiding a direct burn. A modern alternative involves electrifying those needles instead of burning mugwort.

Moxibustion is used to treat stroke, constipation, hypertension, sore muscles, cramps, and menstrual pain. Studies in Japan suggest that it might even prevent breech presentation, which is when babies come out feet first instead of head first. Such studies remain in contention, however.

The smell of burning mugwort also stimulates blood circulation to the pelvic area and uterus, so it's a typical remedy for women who suffer from menstrual cramps and fertility problems. Moxibustion is also used to treat chronic fatigue, lethargy, and mental dullness.

If getting your skin burned is not your thing, watch out for words like *jiǔ* and *jiǔshù* (the formal term for this practice). And if you hear moxibustion being muttered by your doctor, you definitely know what's in store for you. If you're allergic to smoke or have respiratory problems, ask your therapist to use the modern smokeless version.

Chapter 6: Cupping and *Gua Sha*

Sometimes, cupping is also done in tandem with *gua sha*, which literally means scraping. This involves oiling the skin then scraping it with a coin, ceramic spoon, or a scraper made of rhino horn (which is extremely smooth and silky, yet hard) or jade.

This is used to treat fever, exhaustion, sore muscles, and even cellulite. Whatever they use, the skin is scraped along meridian points, which is where the acupoints lie.

In cases of flab, patients lie on their backs while doctors scrape the tummy and/or thighs toward the groin. It's believed this loosens and moves the subcutaneous fat toward the excretory organs for later release.

This treatment causes soreness after a few minutes, and leaves bright red scratch marks on the skin, which fade after 2 to 4 days. Often, the scratches fade long before the bruises from cupping do.

In the 1960s and 1970s, many American doctors wrongly accused Chinese and Vietnamese immigrant parents of child abuse when they discovered these scrapes and cupping bruises on children. Many now understand that this is part of traditional folk remedies, but it's still disturbing to see if you're not used to it.

Gua sha has not yet been medically proven to be an effective form of treatment. Done properly, however, and with sterilized equipment, it can be relaxing except when it comes to treating fat.

In cases of extreme muscle fatigue, such as from hard work or a session at the gym, the scraper is regularly dipped into a solution of ginger root soaked in rice wine or vinegar. It is then used to scrape a person's body from their head, along their spine, and down to their feet.

Odd though this treatment may sound, many swear by it (including the author).

Chapter 7: Cupping and *Tuī Ná*

Tuī means "to push," while *ná* means "to grasp / lift / squeeze." It's a form of massage that's usually done after a cupping session, or after a cupping session but before acupuncture.

Some prefer to call it acupressure, since it's a form of massage that focuses on the acupoints. Unlike Swedish massage which involves rubbing (and some form of oil or cream to make it possible), *tuī ná* focuses on specific points and areas, and rarely makes use of ointments.

Chinese medicine is based on the idea of balance, of symmetry, and of energy streams (known as chi) which flow unobstructed through the body along set paths called meridians. When there is imbalance in the body, then the chi gets blocked, causing illness in areas where the chi can't get to. *Tuī ná* therefore seeks to reopen the blocked passages so that chi can flow through it without problems, restoring harmony throughout the body.

Sometimes, a cupping bruise on the right shoulder (for example) comes out a very dark, almost black color, while the bruise on the left shoulder comes out a healthy, vibrant red. This tells the practitioner that there is an imbalance in the right shoulder or on the right side of the body which needs balancing or unblocking.

Both sides of the body will still be massaged equally to ensure that the chi flows smoothly all over the body. Focusing on only one area could result in an imbalance, further bringing the entire system out of whack.

It is believed that the human body contains eight defensive gates which are located in the area between each joint. When chi is blocked or has difficulty flowing to an area, it not only results in physical illnesses, it can also lead to emotional problems, such as depression, anger, being overly sexed, etc.

A *tuī ná* session is therefore not just about making you feel good, improving your range of motion, as well as getting rid of muscle cramps and stiff joints. It is also about ensuring emotional well-being and improved health by allowing the chi to flow better throughout your body.

It is also believed, however, that a massage is not enough. The acupoints also need to be addressed directly, which is where acupuncture comes in.

Chapter 8: Wet Cupping

This is not used in traditional Chinese medicine, but is popular throughout the Muslim world because the prophet Mohammad recommended it highly in the hadiths (which are interpretations of the Koran). In *Sahih al-Bukhari 5371*, for example, he said that, "Indeed the best of remedies you have is *hijama*."

According to the prophet, wet cupping (*hijama*) is a blessing, a cure or preventative to maintain health and improve memory. It is even said to protect people from black magic, among many others (bearing in mind, of course, that attributing the effect of the magic to anything other than Allah renders one a disbeliever). As such, it isn't always easy to separate fact from fiction, especially under circumstances where an author's belief can sometimes act as a placebo thus rendering his accounts of success unscientific.

Some studies show it to be effective in treating some problems such as migraines, nonspecific lower back pain, and post-herpetic neuralgia. As to its other acclaimed health benefits, on the other hand, those remain in contention. Nevertheless, there are clinics throughout Europe and the Americas which do provide wet cupping services under sterile medical conditions, if you're interested.

Although it requires bleeding, it should be understood that *hijama* is not the same as bloodletting. Bloodletting requires the opening of veins by cutting them with a scalpel, puncturing them with a needle, or by using a leech applied to the skin. *Hijama* extracts blood with tiny incisions to the skin's surface after cupping.

In the UK, the clinics that provide this service make use of sterile plastic cups which are disposed of after each use. The patient's back is first sterilized with alcohol, after which oil is rubbed on the shoulders, as well as the upper and lower back.

The cups are then placed on the skin, after which the air is sucked out from the top with a manual hand pump. The skin is allowed to rise and redden, and after a few minutes, the cups are removed.

Using a surgical scalpel, several tiny incisions are made on the bruised area so that the blood wells up in tiny beads. The cups are then replaced and the practitioner pumps the air out once more, which forces yet more blood to come up. After several minutes, the cups are removed and the blood is wiped away, after which the area is again treated with alcohol.

This is the modern, clinical version, however. If you're interested, you can get in touch with the <u>British Cupping Society</u> for more information.

Since this is a very traditional form of medicine, other practitioners are less clinical and sterile, so this is something you need to watch out for. Because this practice is also deeply associated with religious beliefs, from less scientific records, it is hard to say just how effective it really is, and how much has to do with credulous minds.

That said, there are many who swear by it and undergo regular sessions of hajima. Because the needles or scalpels used are very sharp, it really doesn't hurt too much—more like quick, sharp stings. If done by an expert, no permanent scarring or marks are left behind. Some even believe that regular doses of *hijama* can get rid of old scars, including mild stretch marks, as well as skin discolorations.

Do note, however, that if the area to be wet cupped is hairy, it will be shaved to ensure maximum suction. If you have a hairy back when you go in, you'll leave smooth.

Tradition dictates that hajima be done on an empty stomach, so those undergoing the session are advised to avoid food and drink a full 2 to 3 hours before. You are also advised to avoid strenuous activity for a full 24 hours after. This includes running, swimming, bicycling, and lifting heavy objects. Avoiding a bath a full 24 hours after a session is also recommended to avoid causing the puncture marks to re-open.

Finland also practices wet cupping, which they call *kuppaus*. To avail of it, you have to make your way to a sauna, which is a national obsession. The belief is that the heat of a sauna stimulates better blood flow, making it ideal for wet cupping. For Finns, regular sessions are necessary to get rid of bad blood, release toxins, maintain health and vigor, and avoid more serious illnesses.

After getting baked in steam, you lie face down on a bed. To further stimulate blood circulation, you are gently beaten with a bundle of birch branches called a *vasta*. Your back and legs are then washed, after which they place cups on areas where you feel some aches. If you feel no aches, they'll place them all over anyway.

After a few minutes, they remove the cups and whack the raised spots with a small hammer spiked with pins. Others resort to scalpels. Once the bleeding begins, the cups are returned to draw out more blood. When the bleeding stops, the body and legs are washed and a traditional cream of spruce sap is applied to sterilize the skin. An entire session, from sitting in the sauna to the wet cupping, can take anywhere from 30 minutes to an hour.

In *hijama*, practitioners take special care to avoid letting their patients see their own blood. With the exception of posh resorts which boast such treatments, *kuppaus* sessions are generally quite messy. Some practitioners even make it a point to show patients examples of bad blood, such as thick coagulated clots.

If you want to try wet cupping but are squeamish, therefore, stick to *hijama*.

Chapter 9: A Brief Word about Chinese Medicine

Since traditional Chinese medicine functions on a completely different model than that used by modern medicine, it's only inevitable that certain misunderstandings arise when comparing the two. The same applies when both systems look at the same problem.

Perhaps one of the greatest areas of contention lies in the field of cancer treatments. Barring unscrupulous businesses, misguided professionals, and gullible patients, traditional Chinese medicine has a different understanding of cancer than modern medicine does.

In the former, cancer is not just a disease. It is also a symptom of something else. Sometimes, that something else is an emotional problem, in others it has to do with a digestive imbalance. In treating what it considers to be the root cause, traditional practitioners sometimes claim to have treated the underlying causes of cancer, even though the cancer itself is still present in the patient.

Such claims, therefore, sometimes get taken out of hand or misunderstood outright. Partly, this has to do with the language barrier. Culturally, it also has to do with the fact that traditional doctors try to spare their patients from emotional pain, believing such will only exacerbate the problem.

When the last Japanese Emperor Hirohito died, for example, he wasn't told about his condition, which raised an outcry outside Japan. This puzzled not just the Japanese, but the Chinese, as well. Although modern medical doctors treated the former emperor, they were still Japanese and therefore thought in terms of the old paradigm set by traditional Chinese medicine.

In America, such a practice would be considered deceitful, immoral, outrageous, and deserving of a law suit. It must be understood, however, that we're dealing here with a completely alien psychology, one that plays by a completely different set of rules and values than what we're used to.

At the risk of sounding repetitive, you should therefore consult your GP first before making the final decision about an alternative medical approach.

Conclusion

Cupping, both wet and dry, is an ancient technique still practiced today by millions. Recently, some American and European celebrities have even taken it up, increasing its popularity further.

Dry cupping raises few eyebrows, in addition to the ugly bruises it leaves behind, that is. However, there have been no reports of any complications arising from cupping sessions. As such, it's generally safe, if done properly. There are even home kits that you can buy so you can do it on your own. If you remember the five minute rule and do it no more than twice a week, you should be good to go.

As to wet cupping... well, you're on your own there. Under the right conditions, it can be perfectly safe and can't possibly be worse than some of the other alternative treatments available.

Just be careful, keep an open mind, and once again—consult your GP.

Finally, I'd like to thank you for purchasing this book! If you found it helpful, I'd greatly appreciate it if you'd take a moment to leave a review on Amazon. Thank you!

Made in the USA
San Bernardino, CA
12 September 2016